C000048166

UROLOGY FOR MEDICAL STUDENTS AND JUNIOR DOCTORS

Written by

RICKY ELLIS

Specialist Registrar in Urology

Edited by

Giacomo Caddeo

Consultant Urological Surgeon, University Hospitals of Derby and Burton NHS Foundation Trust

Dhaval Bodiwala

Consultant Urological Surgeon, Nottingham University Hospitals

Sharon Scriven

Consultant Urological Surgeon, Nottingham University Hospitals

Illustration and cover art by

Giacomo Caddeo

Consultant Urological Surgeon, University Hospitals of Derby and Burton NHS Foundation Trust

ISBN 979-8-6432-6326-5

Contents

1. Foreword

To all medical students, the aim of this book is to help you gain a better understanding of Urology and its key principles. I often hear students telling me that they feel Urology is brushed over in their training and I for one felt this way throughout my studies. Urology is an expanding speciality and certainly one that you will deal with no matter which area of medicine you dedicate your career to. You will almost definitely have to deal with urological pathology when working as a junior doctor and this can be incredibly daunting if you have had limited exposure to the speciality as a student. With a good base of knowledge and some practical tips I hope that you will feel a little more comfortable in the acute management of these conditions.

It is important to remember as you go through your training that every doctor throughout history has been in your position, once again faced with the overwhelming prospect of having to learn yet another medical speciality. I vividly remember wondering how on earth I was going to remember everything for my final exams! It helps to remember that you are not just studying in order to pass your medical school examinations; you are studying to become a good, safe and confident doctor.

To all junior doctors, I understand how out of your depth you can feel when rotating from one speciality to another with a new set of expectations weighing heavily on you every time. A lot of responsibility is placed on your shoulders, even as the most junior member of the team, but remember that we provide the best care for our patients when working together. Ask your colleagues and seniors for advice, find mentors to learn from and utilise the wealth of experience and knowledge of others around you. Over time try and give a little back to the next generation of doctors where possible.

I created this book in an effort to try and give back to yourselves, tomorrow's doctors and to help teach a subject which I felt was too often overlooked in my early training. It is my sincere hope that this book will help you to understand Urology in a way that is easier for you to remember for both your exams and when working as a junior doctor. I hope that this can become a quick reference guide for you that is easily accessible on your mobile devices and tablets whenever you come across a urological problem and are in need of some advice. Please remember to leave a review of the book and tell your colleagues about it so that it can help others too.

In purchasing this book you are also raising money for charity, so a big thankyou for your support.

I wish you all luck and look forward to working with you in the future.

Ricky Ellis

2. Urological Emergencies

2.1 Haematuria

Haematuria is the presence of blood in the urine. It is one of the most common presenting complaints in urology and can be a sign of many urological conditions. We categorise it into either **visible** (macroscopic) or **non-visible** (microscopic) haematuria. Non-visible is picked up on urine dipstick testing or mid-stream urine sampling.

You will often hear haematuria being described rather crudely by urologists as looking like Rosé wine, Merlot or Ribena. Although it's not ideal to draw comparison between your patients urine with what may be your favourite tipple it is a rather handy way of describing the severity of haematuria to the on-call urologist and this description may even change the immediate management of the patient.

Non-visible haematuria or light Rosé coloured visible haematuria can be investigated as an outpatient according to the NICE guidelines below. However, darker haematuria will likely require admission for inpatient management.

When to refer to Urology for review within 2 weeks: NICE Guidelines

2 Week wait referral if <u>aged 45</u> and over and have:

- Unexplained <u>visible</u> haematuria without urinary tract infection **or**
- Visible haematuria that persists or recurs after successful treatment of urinary tract infection, **or**
- Aged 60 and over and have unexplained <u>nonvisible haematuria</u> **and** either dysuria or a raised white cell count on a blood test

Consider non-urgent referral for bladder cancer in people aged 60 and over with recurrent or persistent unexplained urinary tract infection.

We will discuss the signs and symptoms of each individual cause of haematuria in later chapters, but for now let's look at the questions you would like to ask in your history:

Some common causes of haematuria

Kidneys
- Pelvi-Calyceal (e.g. Transitional cell carcinoma, Stones)
- Pre-renal (e.g. Clotting disorders, Rhabdomyolysis (myoglobinuria))
- Renal (e.g. Glomerulonephritis, Acute tubular necrosis, Henoch Schonlein Purpura, Cancer, Trauma)

Ureters
- Transitional cell carcinoma, Stones

Bladder
- Transitional cell carcinoma, Other cancers, Stones, Cystitis, Radiation cystitis, UTI

Prostate
- Malignancy, Benign prostatic enlargement, Prostatitis

Urethra
- Transitional cell carcinoma, Trauma

Vagina
- Always rule out bleeding from the vagina as a cause

Pseudo-haematuria
- e.g. beetroot, rifampicin

2. Urological Emergencies

- Presenting complaint and History of presenting complaint
- When did it start?
- Change in colour over time?
- Clots in the urine?
- Mixed with urine or separate?
- Timing of onset with micturition (i.e. continuous or just at the start/end of micturition)
- Painful vs painless
- Abdominal or flank pain
- Symptoms of anaemia
- Weight loss/ fatigue/ Night sweats and other red flag symptoms
- Past medical history
- Medication (e.g. anti-coagulants, prostate medications, rifampicin, chemotherapy e.g. cyclophosphamide) etc.
- Family and Social history including: occupation, smoking status and travel History

How would you manage significant visible haematuria initially?

- Assess acutely unwell patients according to the principles of Advanced life support (see ALS manual in references): **ABCDE** (**A**irway, **B**reathing, **C**irculation, **D**isability, **E**verything else). The principles of an ABCDE assessment and the initial management of an acutely unwell patient lie outside the remit of this revision book, however they can be found in all Advanced life support text books. These principles should be thoroughly understood as you will rely on them as a junior doctor to provide a thorough, systematic and safe assessment of an unwell patient.
- Apply oxygen
- Intravenous (IV) access
- Bloods (including a full blood count, renal function, clotting, plus consider a group and save etc.)
- Fluid (+/- Blood) resuscitation as required
- **3-way** Catheter
- Mid-stream/Catheter urine sample
- Take a full history
- Examine the patient
- Admit the patient and inform your senior
- Consider starting continuous irrigation of the bladder via the 3 way catheter +/- bladder washouts on the ward. In cases of haematuria, the sooner this is done the better. A prompt 3-way catheter and irrigation can potentially prevent clot formation within the bladder and reduce the risk of needing an emergency bladder washout in theatre.

Further investigation of haematuria

- Imaging of the upper tracts
- Flexible cystoscopy

As a general rule, all patients with haematuria will require imaging of the upper urinary tracts and a cystoscopic examination of the bladder.

The two most common imaging modalities used to visualise the upper tracts are an **ultrasound scan** of the kidneys, ureters and bladder or a **CT scan** with contrast.

The advantage of ultrasound is that its fast to obtain, does not expose the patient to radiation and is possible no matter what the patients' renal function is, making it an ideal imaging modality to use in the first instance. However, it is user and recipient dependant and it is possible to miss small tumours or stones.

CT scans have a greater sensitivity and specificity although they involve radiation and may involve contrast which can worsen renal function and can lead to anaphylaxis. Therefore you should check with your seniors before you order a CT scan to ensure that it is indicated for that patient. In the case of haematuria we often ask for a CT Urogram, this is a scan which is taken in a delayed phase after the intravenous contrast has been given in order to visualise the urinary tract as the contrast highlights the kidneys, ureters and bladder.

Of all patients suffering with visible haematuria, 1 in 5 will have an underlying bladder cancer. 1 in 12 patients exhibiting non-visible haematuria will have underlying bladder cancer. Kidney, prostate or ureteric cancer is found in approximately 1% of all patients referred with haematuria.

2.2 Acute urinary retention (AUR)

An acute cessation of urinary flow resulting in a painful distended bladder. This will often present with anuria and supra pubic pain which can be severe.

Acute vs chronic retention

- Acute will generally be painful, whilst chronic is generally painless
- Chronic retention will often be of very large volumes
- Chronic will be an insidious onset, often with a long history of LUTS

In practice, you often find cases of acute-on-chronic retention. In these cases patients often describe a history of progressive LUTS followed by going into acute painful retention as a result of a precipitating event e.g. UTI or surgery.

Signs and symptoms

- Difficulty passing urine
- Abdominal/Suprapubic pain
- Restlessness
- Possible preceeding lower urinary tract symptoms
- May have suffered with dysuria or haematuria or constipation prior to retention

Examination findings may include

- Tenderness suprapubically
- May have a palpable bladder
- Enlarged or abnormal prostate on digital rectal examination
- Always check for neurological abnormalities and rule out cauda equina syndrome

Things to ask in your history:

- Presenting complaint and history of presenting complaint
- Duration
- Acute or more insidious onset?
- Painful vs painless retention?
- Urinary symptoms prior to onset?
  - Lower urinary tract symptoms (LUTS) we will discuss these later in chapter *5.1*
  - Haematuria, dysuria
- Systemic symptoms (e.g. infection, constipation)
- Other precipitants e.g. alcohol, recent surgery (especially abdominal), acute pain
- Previous Urological history
- Red flag symptoms
- Past medical history
- Medication (e.g. phenilephrine, anti-cholinergics, prostate medications)
- Systematic review
- Then perform a thorough investigation including the abdomen, external genitalia and a digital rectal examination
- Rule out Cauda Equina syndrome

Some common causes of urinary retention

Urological

- Benign prostatic enlargement
- Blocked catheter
- Failed trial without a catheter (TWOC)
- Clot retention
- Prostate/ bladder/ urethral cancer
- Urethral stricture

Gastrointestinal

- Constipation
- Infection
- Malignancy
- Inflammatory bowel disease (UC, Crohns)
- Surgery

Systemic

- Infection
- Pain

Medication

- Phenylephrine, anti-cholinergics

Neuro

- Multiple sclerosis, Guillain-Barré, Spinal Cord injury, Cauda Equina Syndrome etc.

How would you manage AUR initially?

- Assess according to the principles of ALS (ABCDE)
- IV Access
- Bloods (including full blood count and renal function)
- Fluid resuscitation
- Catheter (2-way catheter 14-16Fr unless there is a history of haematuria in which case consider inserting a 3-way catheter)
- Record the residual volume that drains from the catheter
- Send a Catheter Urine sample
- Take a full history
- Examine the patient
- Inform your senior
- Monitor for diuresis and replace fluid loses if needed. If diuresis occurs discuss with on call urologist
- Monitor electrolytes (and haemoglobin if haematuria present)

How you manage this afterwards will depend entirely on the cause of retention. All reversible causes should be optimised prior to performing a trial without a catheter. If there is a history or LUTS, the patient may require an alpha-blocker such as tamsulosin to help them pass their TWOC and improve their symptoms. A urological opinion should be sought to help guide the long term management of these patients.

If the patient has a large residual volume of urine (>1L) or deranged renal function (high-creatinine) this may indicate high-pressure chronic retention. In these cases the urologist will send the patient home with a catheter in situ until they undergo definitive treatment for their bladder outflow obstruction. Patients with high-pressure chronic retention will need admitting for observation overnight. It is common for these patients to develop significant diuresis after catheterisation, and some may develop a degree of haematuria as the bladder is decompressed. In most cases this diuresis will settle over 24-48 hours but the patient may require careful fluid management over this time which will require input from the urology team.

Acute urinary retention in females occurs less frequently. It is imperative that neurological causes of retention are ruled out in females presenting with AUR. Other causes usually involve obstruction of the urethra (e.g. stricture, surgery for stress incontinence or compression due to gynaecological pathology such as fibroids, ovarian mass/cysts or prolapse).

2.3 Testicular torsion

When the spermatic cord twists cutting off the blood supply to the testicle resulting in ischaemic necrosis and possibly the loss of the testicle.

Differential diagnoses for acute scrotal pain include: epididymo-orchitis and torted hydatid of Morgagni.

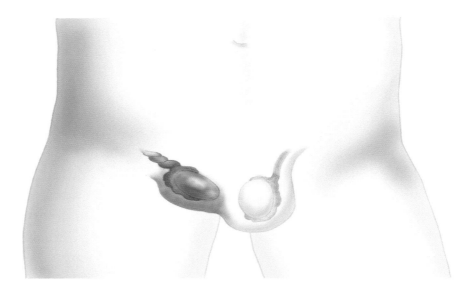

Figure 1: Testicular torsion. Here the right testicle is twisted on its blood supply, causing ischaemia. It is high riding and has a transverse lie when compared to the normal left testicle.

Signs and symptoms	• Sudden onset testicular pain • May radiate to the back/loin • Most common in 10-30 years of age but can occur at any age including prepubertal children • Can be associated with local trauma • May have had a self resolving episode of groin pain (though not as severe) sometime before this started • Nausea and Vomiting
Examination findings may include	• Extremely tender testicle • High riding, fixed testicle • Abnormal, horizontal lie of the testicle • Swelling • Discolouration of the scrotal skin • Note: Blue dot sign in children is an indication of a torted hydatid of Morgagni • Absent cremasteric reflex

2. Urological Emergencies

- Time of onset of pain?
- Has it changed over time?
- Any radiation of pain?
- Full pain history (see pain history box below)
- Trauma?
- History of similar episodes?
- Recent unprotected sexual intercourse?
- Sexual health history
- Penile discharge?
- Dysuria?
- Fever?
- LUTS discussed in chapter **5.1**
- Urinary tract infections
- Recent instrumentation/catheterisation of the urinary tract?
- Urological history or previous scrotal surgery?

How to take a pain history:

- Site
- Onset
- Character
- Radiation
- Associated symptoms
- Time course
- Exacerbating/Relieving factors
- Severity

How would you manage testicular torsion initially?

- Assess according to the principles of ALS (ABCDE)
- Apply oxygen
- IV Access
- Bloods (including full blood count, renal function, CRP, clotting)
- Fluid resuscitation if required
- Take a full history
- Examine the patient
- Urine dipstick (signs of infection may point towards epididymo-orchitis as a differential diagnosis of this acute testicular pain)
- Inform your senior ASAP
- Keep patient nil by mouth
- +/- Make theatre and anaesthetic teams aware
- Do you perform an Ultrasound of the testes?
  - NO! You would only perform this if it is requested by the Urologist. Ultrasound scans cannot definitively rule out a testicular torsion and therefore waste valuable time – the patient needs to go to theatre for exploration!

What do we do in theatre for a torted testicle? We perform an exploration of the scrotum, untwist the testicle, wrap it in warm saline soaked gauze to see if it re-perfuses. If it does not after waiting then an **orchidectomy** is required (removal of the testicle) as it is non-viable. If it reperfuses then **orchidopexy** (fixation of the testes in the scrotum) is performed, bilaterally.

2.4 The obstructed infected kidney

An obstructed infected kidney can result in the rapid development of urosepsis and septic shock. It can also result in the loss of kidney function and is often extremely painful for patients; therefore it is imperative that it is picked up early. The most common cause of an obstructed infected kidney is a stone that has popped out of the kidney and has started to travel down the ureter towards the bladder. They commonly get stuck at one of 3 locations: the pelvi-ureteric junction (at the very top of the ureter), as the ureter crosses the iliac vessels or at the vesico-ureteric junction (at the very bottom of the ureter).

An obstructed kidney will result in urinary stasis which may harbour infection, it also increases intra-renal pressures which can cause renal damage, therefore it is important that we find a way of draining the kidney quickly if it is infected and obstructed.

Things to ask in your history:

- Presenting complaint and history of presenting complaint
- Systematic pain history
- Onset of symptoms
- Previous episodes
- Any known stones?
- Previous Urological problems
- Recurrent urinary tract infections?
- Red flag symptoms
- Family History
- Social History
- Fluid intake history
- Follow with a thorough examination

Signs and symptoms of an infected obstructed kidney may include

- Fever
- Rigors
- Loin-groin/back/abdominal pain
- Haematuria
- Tachycardia
- Tachypnoea
- High early warning score (NEWS)
- Other sequelae of sepsis e.g. hypotension, atrial fibrillation, reduced urine output etc

How would you manage an infected obstructed kidney initially?

- Assess according to the principles of ALS (ABCDE) and Sepsis 6
- Apply oxygen
- IV Access
- Bloods (including blood Cultures x2, lactate, full blood count, renal function, CRP, urate and calcium)
- Fluid resuscitation and maintenance
- Urine dipstick and send sample for culture and sensitivities
- Pregnancy test
- Assess urine output and fluid status
- Start antibiotics according to previous recent sensitivities, if not available then follow local guidelines
- Admit the patient and inform your senior ASAP
- Keep patient nil by mouth unless told otherwise
- Imaging (unless contra-indicated a CT KUB is usually an ideal imaging modality to look for an obstructing stone)

We have two temporary treatment options for draining an infected obstructing kidney.

1. The first temporary procedure is the insertion of a **Ureteric stent** (also known as a **JJ Stent**). This is performed in theatre and involves the placement of a flexible tube in the ureter which coils in the kidney and coils in the bladder to hold it in place. The urine is then able to drain through and around the stent into the bladder.

2. The second temporary procedure is the insertion of a **Nephrostomy**. This is similar to the JJ stent but the tube passes through the skin on the patient's back/flank directly into the kidney to drain urine from the kidney into a bag which is stuck to the patient's skin.

Once the infected kidney has been drained with one of the above treatments the patient can undergo definitive treatment of the stone at a later date. We will cover treatment options for kidney and ureteric stones in Chapter *3.3*.

2.5 Urological Trauma

Renal Trauma

Renal trauma is not uncommon and can be classified as either penetrative or blunt trauma. Common causes of penetrative trauma to the kidneys include stab and gunshot wounds. Blunt trauma are however far more common and includes road traffic accidents, falls, assault and contact sports etc.

<table>
<tr>
<td>Signs and symptoms of renal trauma may include</td>
<td>

•A suspicious mechanism of injury
•Possible haematuria
•Loin or back pain
•Haemodynamic instability
•Damage to surrounding structures e.g. ribs, vertebrae, spleen, bowel

</td>
</tr>
</table>

Despite renal injuries appearing to be severe, there are relatively few indications for surgical exploration and treatment. All require contrast enhanced CT scans to visualise the extent of the injury and will require and urgent Urology review, but most patients do very well with conservative management which includes a period of close observation and bed rest.

Ureteric Trauma

By far the most common cause of damage to the ureters is iatrogenic injury. Ureters are small in diameter and can be hard to identify in difficult intra-abdominal operations. Ureters can also be damaged by urologists performing ureteroscopy (the insertion of a very long pointy scope up the ureters) and when fragmenting stones with a laser in the ureter.

Signs and symptoms of ureteric trauma may include	• Suspicious mechanism of injury • Insidious onset of generalised symptoms which may include: • Peritonitis • Abdominal Pain • Ileus • Urinoma (collection of urine) • Urine leaking from wound or a fistula

If a ureteric injury is suspected; a urologist should be consulted immediately.

Bladder trauma

Bladder trauma can also be classified into either penetrative or blunt trauma. The most common cause of penetrative trauma is iatrogenic (often caused during resection of bladder tumours or whilst performing intra-abdominal or pelvic operations). The bladder is at high risk of injury in all pelvic fractures so have a high level of suspicion in pelvic crush injuries, road traffic accidents, including seat belt injury after a night in the pub and high impact falls.

Signs and symptoms of bladder trauma may include	• Suspicious mechanism of injury • Pelvic fractures (urethra may be injured as well) • Peritonism • Abdominal distension • Ileus • Oliguric/anuric • Haematuria • Blood at the urethral meatus • Perineal/scrotal bruising • High riding prostate

When a bladder injury is suspected only urologists or senior clinicians should be making a single attempt at gentle catheterisation. A CT scan with contrast or a cystogram is often used to diagnose a perforation and to identify its location within the bladder. If the perforation is extraperitoneal a urethral catheter is placed for 2-3 weeks to allow the bladder to heal. If the perforation is intraperitoneal then open surgical repair is required.

Penile Fracture

Rupture of the tunica albuginea whilst the penis is erect (one or both of the corpora cavernosa and possibly the corpora spongiosum which may include rupture of the urethra).

Signs and symptoms of a penile fracture may include	• Feeling of a 'snap' or 'pop' whilst the penis is erect • Followed by immediate detumescence • The penis has a characteristic 'eggplant' appearance which includes • Swelling • Discolouration due to bruising • Defomity towards the area of injury to the tunica

This requires urgent urological review and surgical repair in an attempt to preserve erectile function.

2.6 Paraphimosis

Paraphimosis describes when the foreskin is retracted behind the glans and cannot be replaced again resulting in a tight ring of tissue around the corona. This is an emergency and is not to be mistaken with 'phimosis' (a tight foreskin which is difficult to retract).

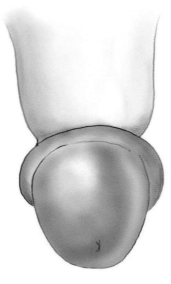

Figure 2: Paraphimosis. Here you can see the foreskin has retracted behind the corona of glans penis, forming a tight band. This will lead to venous occlusion, congestive oedema and will eventually compromise the blood supply to the glans and foreskin, causing ischaemia.

Signs and symptoms of paraphimosis may include

- Foreskin retracted behind the corona of glans penis
- Penile oedema
- Possible discolouration (a sign of ischaemia) and even necrosis
- Cracks in the skin
- Some may be painful, others go unnoticed by the patient
- Commonly seen in catheterised patients

Paraphimosis occurs when an already phimotic (tight) foreskin is retracted past the glans and is not returned to its normal position. This is also commonly caused iatrogenically, when the foreskin is not replaced to its original position after catheterisation.

Paraphimosis requires urgent reduction. If left alone, the tight band of tissue around the corona will cause venous congestion leading to oedema of the tissues which can result in arterial occlusion and ischaemic necrosis.

There are various different ways to reduce a paraphimosis. These all aim to reduce the swelling in the tissues to enable you to replace the foreskin to its original position. All methods will reduce swelling a little and aided with gentle pressure on the distal tissue prior to reduction of the foreskin most cases of paraphimosis can be successfully treated in a prompt fashion. It is relatively rare that the patient would require emergency surgical intervention.

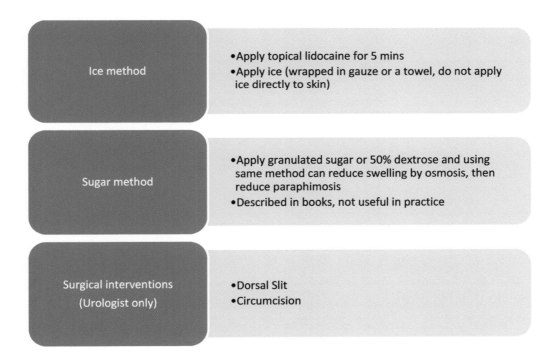

Ice method
- Apply topical lidocaine for 5 mins
- Apply ice (wrapped in gauze or a towel, do not apply ice directly to skin)

Sugar method
- Apply granulated sugar or 50% dextrose and using same method can reduce swelling by osmosis, then reduce paraphimosis
- Described in books, not useful in practice

Surgical interventions (Urologist only)
- Dorsal Slit
- Circumcision

Once reduced all patients should be followed up by the urology team as a circumcision will likely be required to prevent this occurring again in the future.

2.7 Fournier's Gangrene

Necrotising fasciitis of the genitalia and perineum. Fournier's Gangrene is a urological emergency, the mortality rate is upwards of 20%, more so if a patient is immunocompromised. The infection spreads rapidly along fascial planes causing necrosis and gangrene. It is a synergistic infection caused by a combination of both aerobic and anaerobic organisms. Aerobic organisms involved often include *E.Coli, Klebsiella,* or *Enterococci,* and common anaerobic organisms can include *Clostridium* or *Bacteroides.*

Signs and symptoms of Fournier's Gangrene may include	•Acutely unwell patient •Sepsis •Erythematous tender area around the external genitalia or perineum (ensure a thorough examination is performed including under the scrotum) •Blistering of the skin •Crepitus (causes by gas-forming organisms) •Discolouration or the area as necrosis occurs, turning blue/black

Risk Factors

- Diabetes Mellitus
- Catheterisation or instrumentation of the urethra
- Immunocompromise
- Post-surgery
- Perineal and peri-anal infections
- Steroid therapy

How would you manage Fournier's Gangrene initially?

- Assess according to the principles of ALS (ABCDE) and Sepsis 6
- Apply oxygen
- IV Access
- Bloods (including blood Cultures x2, lactate, full blood count, renal function, CRP, group and save)
- Fluid resuscitation and maintenance
- Start broad-spectrum antibiotics immediately in accordance with microbiology advice and local hospital guidelines
- Alert the Urologist on-call immediately
- Keep patient nil by mouth
- Make anaesthetist and theatre team aware
- Make ITU aware as will likely require higher level of care after theatre
- Make general surgical team aware if involving the perineum
- Urology team will take patient to theatre immediately to debride necrotic tissue

2.8 Priapism

"The persistence of an unwanted erection for more than 4 hours in the absence of sexual stimulation."

The longer priapism is left untreated the more likely it is that the patient will suffer with erectile dysfunction following the episode.

Priapism can be broken down into **3 types**:

Low flow priapism

- Also known as Ischaemic priapism
- This is caused by venous occlusion, resulting in a rigid, painful erection.
- If aspirated the intracavernosal blood would be acidotic with a low pO2, a high pCO2 and a high lactate.
- This is an emergency and requires immediate escalation to the Urologist on call.

High flow priapism

- Also known as Arterial priapism
- This is caused by dysfunctional arterial flow resulting in a semi-rigid, painless erection.
- The patient will often give a history of trauma which results in the formation of an arteriovenous fistula.

Recurrent Priapism

- Also known as Stuttering priapism.
- It is most commonly seen in patients with sickle cell disease.
- Often painful and self-limiting but can turn into episodes of low flow priapism.

Things to ask in your history:

- When did it start?
- Is it painful?
- Has there been any trauma or surgery to the area?
- Has this occurred before?
- If so how was this treated previously?
- Past medical history: e.g. sickle cell disease, haematological problems, spinal cord pathology
- Medications (e.g. treatments for erectile dysfunction, TPN)
- Have they taken any recreational drugs?

Management of Priapism

Low Flow

- Inform the urologist on call immediately.
- On presentation the patient can try exercise (ask them to climb a few flights of stairs if possible) and cooling the area with ice packs.
- If this fails the penis should be aspirated by the urologist on call using large gauge cannulas or butterfly needles.
- If this fails intracavernosal injection of an α1-adrenergic agonist (phenylephrine) can be given by the urologist under cardiac monitoring in an appropriate setting (e.g. resus or recovery bays) with a support team present.
- If detumescence is still not achieved the patient will need to go to theatre for a shunt procedure to be performed.
- Following this there is a high chance of erectile dysfunction; therefore these patients will likely require referral to a specialist centre for insertion of a penile prosthesis.

High Flow

- This can often be managed conservatively, but if intervention is required then this is often in the form of selective embolization of the supplying arteries.

Recurrent

- If sickle cell disease: Hyperhydration, hyperoxygenation, haematological optimisation and analgesia.

3. Renal pathology

3.1 Congenital Abnormalities

Pelvic Ureteric Junction Obstruction (PUJO)

- Many causes
- A narrowing in the ureter as it joins Renal Pelvis
- Obstructs flow of urine from kidney
- Increased risk of Infections, stones, renal failure
- Can present with hydronephrosis in childhood or adulthood
- Sometimes causes loin pain/discomfort

Horseshoe kidney

- Kidneys fuse to form one big kidney
- The part that joins them is called the isthmus
- What consequences may this cause?
  - Often don't ascend high enough as unable to pass the Inferior Mesenteric Artery
  - Increased risk of kidney stones, pyelonephritis (reflux) and PUJ obstruction

Renal Agenesis and Dysplasia

- Often unilateral
- Kidney is either absent or underdeveloped
- Often an obstructive component if dysplastic

Renal Cysts

- Increase in frequency with age
- Rarely affect renal function
- Observe if simple cysts but if a scan suggests that a cyst is complex, it will require further imaging to rule out malignancy

Adult Polycystic Kidneys

- Commonly causes chronic kidney disease
- Lots of cysts throughout both kidneys
- Increased risk of hepatic and pancreatic cysts, hypertension, intracranial aneurisms, valve abnormalities (especially mitral valve prolapse)

Ectopic Kidney

- Kidney ascends insufficiently
- Increased risk of PUJO
- Commonly found in the pelvis
- Some are non-functioning

3.2 Renal Cancer

These can be symptomatic or found incidentally on Ultrasound scans or CT scans. There are several types of renal cancer, the most common ones that you need to know are:

Renal Cell Carcinoma

- Commonest renal tumour (85%).
- Male:Female = 1.5 : 1
- Adenocarcinoma.
- 50% 5 year survival.
- 1-2% Bilateral.
- Average age 60-70.

Transitional Cell Carcinoma

- Originates from urothelial cells anywhere along urinary tract.
- Male:Female = 3:1
- Make up 10% renal tumours.

Wilms Tumour (Nephroblastoma)

- Commonest intra-abdominal tumour in children
- 1:10,000.
- Male:Female.
- 20% Familial.
- 5% Bilateral.

Risk Factors

Smoking

- 1.4-2.3 fold risk

CKD and Dialysis

- 30 fold risk

HTN

- 1.4-2 fold risk

Male:Female ratio

- 2:1

Obesity

Age

Hereditary

- Von-Hippel Lindau (VHL)
- Hereditary papillary renal cell carcinoma (HPRCC)
- Hereditary non-polyposis colorectal cancer (HNPCC)
- Birt-Hogg-Dube (BHD)
- Hereditary leiomyoma renal cell carcinoma
- Cowden syndrome
- Tuberous Sclerosis

Signs and symptoms of kidney cancer may include	• A mass (especially in Wilms tumours)
	• Haematuria
	• Loin pain
	• Hypertension
	• Signs of metastatic spread
	• Left Sided Varicocele
	  • Involvement of Left Renal vein causes obstruction of left testicular vein. Whereas the right spermatic vein drains directly into IVC
	• Paraneoplastic Syndromes
	  • E.g. Polycythaemia (Due to paraneoplastic erythropoietin production)
	  • Anaemia
	  • Hypertension
	  • Hypercalcaemia due to excretion of PTH related hormone
	  • Abnormal LFT's fue to Stauffers syndrome

Note: Fewer than 10% of patients present with the 'classic triad' of a mass, haematuria and pain.
    (Most renal tumours are identified incidentally on imaging)

- Haematuria
- Loin/back/abdominal pain (full pain history if so)
- Palpable lump in flank/abdomen
- Red Flags
  - Weight loss
  - Bone pain
  - Night sweats
  - Fatigue
  - Loss of appetite
  - Haemoptysis
- Past medical history
  - Chronic kidney disease (CKD)
  - Anaemia
  - Dialysis
  - Hypertension
  - Known congenital abnormailities
- Social history
  - Smoking
  - Occupation
- Family History

When answering any question on the management of a chronic disease, always try to categorise your answer. I have always used the following categories to aim for a holistic and stepwise approach to managing the patient:

Management of kidney cancer

Psychosocial factors

- Macmillan support, cancer specialist nurse support, lifestyle factors, support at home. All of these will be tailored to the patient's individual needs.

Medical

- Active surveillance
  - Sometimes we keep a close eye on a small suspicious lesion and only intervene if it becomes symptomatic or grows to a significant size.
- Radiotherapy (though renal cell carcinoma are radio-resistant)
- Chemotherapy
- Palliative therapy

Surgical (these can be performed as open operations, laparoscopically or robot-assisted)

- Radical nephrectomy
- Partial nephrectomy
- Nephrouretectomy (for transitional cell carcinoma, the ureter is taken with the kidney)
- Renal artery embolisation (usually if unfit for surgery and refractory haematuria)

3.3 Kidney Stones

These are very common so you are highly likely to diagnose a fair few in your career. A renal colic history is also quite common place in medical school examinations. On average 1 in 10 will get kidney stones and the risk is even higher for those who have previously developed stones.

These can be diagnosed using a number of imaging modalities. **X-Ray** of the kidneys, ureters and bladder (KUB) can be useful although only 60-70% of stones are radio-opaque and therefore it is possible to miss some on x-ray. Additionally, large body habitus and overlying bowel gas can degrade image quality. **Ultrasound** KUB can be useful in detecting renal stones and hydronephrosis, but it may struggle to see small stones and stones in the ureters, therefore it is not the ideal imaging modality to use in cases of acute colic. You may hear of **Intravenous Urograms** being used where we give the patient radio-opaque contrast and watch it drain through the urinary tract using X-Rays to look for filling defects and obstruction, that may represent a stone. However these are largely obsolete these days due to improved CT imaging techniques.

The gold standard investigation to assess the first presentation of renal colic is therefore a **CT KUB**. This is a non-contrast, low dose CT which is able to pick up almost 100% of stones. It is non-contrast so you need not worry about a patient's renal function or risk of contrast allergy. They are also quick scans that are easy to perform and are therefore readily available in an acute setting.

From a CT KUB you can assess the size and location of the stone, how hard the stone is (by measurement of Hounsfield units), and whether there are any signs of the stone having blocked the ureter causing obstruction of urinary flow from the kidney (often presenting on the scan as hydronephrosis (swollen kidney). You can also rule out a ruptured abdominal aortic aneurysm which is an extremely important differential diagnosis to consider when anyone presents with acute onset back/ abdominal/ loin/ loin-to-groin pain.

What signs and symptoms may make you consider renal colic as a differential diagnosis warranting further investigation?

Signs and symptoms of renal colic may include	• Loin or loin-to-groin pain • Often described as the worst pain they have ever felt • Cannot sit still (the opposite of when a patient is peritonitic) • Associated nausea, clammy • Tachycardia • Haematuria (visible or non-visible)

Signs and symptoms of infection may include	• Pyrexial • Tachycardia • Tachypnoea • Inflammatory markers raised • Sequelae of infection such as atrial fibrillation • Etc.

There are several different types of stones that can form in the urinary tract. I have tried to summarise them for you in the table below.

Stone Composition	% of all Renal Calculi	Cause	Radiodensity
Calcium Oxalate	80-85	Acidic urine	Radio-opaque
Uric acid	5-10	Acidic urine	Radio-Lucent
Struvite	2-20	Kidney infections	Radio-opaque
Cystine	1	Genetic	Slightly radio-opaque
Calcium Phosphate	Rare	Alkaline urine Hyperparathyroidism	Radio-opaque

There are many predisposing factors to stone formation. Some of these are listed below. I have categorised them into intrinsic and extrinsic factors and have briefly explained why they predispose an individual to forming urinary calculi. In essence, the cause of urinary stones is supersaturation of the urine with one or more of the components which form stones.

Intrinsic Factors

Age

- Peak incidence = 20 - 50yrs

Sex (Male:Female = approximately 1.5 : 1)

- Males: Testosterone causes increased oxalate production -> predisposing to calcium oxalate stones
- Females: Higher urinary citrate -> which inhibits calcium oxalate stone formation. Also have a predisposition to UTI's increasing the risk of Struvite stones.

Genetics

- Increased risk in caucasian and asian populations
- Family history of stones
- Familial renal tubular acidosis (calcium phosphate stones)
- Cystinuria (cystine stones)
- Primary Hyperoxaluria (Ca Oxalate stones)
- Hypercalcuria (many causes of this which include hyperparathyroidism)
- Hyperuricaemia (gout, myeloproliferative disorders)

Anatomical abnormalities

- Horseshoe/ duplex kidney
- PUJO
- Anything that causes urinary stasis/ delayed emptying

Urinary tract infections

- Urease hydrolyses urea to ammonium raising urine pH

Medication

- E.g. Loop diuretics and steroids (calcium stones), chemotherapy (hyperuricaemia)
- Anti-epileptics e.g. Topiramate

Extrinsic Factors

Geography

- Western lifestyle
- Hot climates

Fluid intake

- <1.2L/day is a risk

Occupation

- Sedentary lifestyle
- Working in hot environments e.g. kitchens

Diet

- High Protein = Excessive purine excretion causing uric acid stones
- High Salt = Hypercalciuria
- Low calcium = Higher risk of calcium stones which I agree is not as you would expect!
- Malabsorptive diseases: hyperoxaluria (reduced binding of calcium = increased absorption of oxalate)

We have already discussed how to manage acute colic in chapter *2.4*. However, many renal stones can be managed on an elective basis, the indications for **emergency** intervention are:

1. Signs of infection

2. A single functioning kidney

3. Renal Impairment

4. Obstruction of the kidney

5. Other factors taking patient into account (e.g. previous ITU admissions due to stones etc.)

How could we manage the patient if they have one of the above?

As discussed in chapter *2.4* we need to drain the kidney as soon as possible. Consider either:

- JJ Stent
- Nephrostomy
- Primary treatment of the stone

The patient has none of the indications for emergency intervention, what are the options for treatment of the stone?

Management of stones

Conservative management

- Often stones can pass on their own depending on their size. The patient will require analgesia, reassurance and a follow up scan to check whether the stone has passed a few weeks later. Sometimes alpha-blockers such as tamsulosin may be given in an attempt to expedite stone passage. The patient must be given safety netting advice which should include instructions to return to A+E immediately if they develop the signs or symptoms of an infected obstructed kidney or if their symptoms worsen. If the stone is less than 4mm in size the patient has over 80% chance of passing it spontaneously over the next 30 days!

Extracorporeal shockwave lithotripsy (ESWL)

- Performed in a dedicated clinic with analgesia. We use shock waves to fragment the stone into smaller pieces which the patient will hopefully be able to pass spontaneously.

Ureteroscopy and stone fragmentation

- Performed in theatre under an anaesthetic. A very long but thin endoscope is passed via the urethra into the bladder then up into the ureter and into the kidney. With this scope we can use a number of devices such as laser to fragment the stone, we can then remove the fragments with small baskets passed through the scope.

Percutaneous nephrolithotomy (PCNL)

- A tube is placed through the skin into the kidney under radiological guidance. We can then use this tube to insert a scope into the kidney and fragment the stones, removing fragments. This is still a minimally invasive procedure with only a small cut in the skin but it can be used to remove larger stones from the kidney.

Open nephrolithotomy

- Rarely performed now in countries with endoscopic equipment available. Performed for large staghorn stones in specific cases.

Medical dissolution therapy

- Can be used to treat uric acid stones (where the aim is to alkalinise the urine) and cystine stones (aim is to alkalinise the urine and also reduce dietary intake).

With this many options available for the treatment of stones, things can get relatively confusing. I have therefore attempted to simplify the treatment of stones in the following table, although keep in mind that treatment may vary depending on the patient.

Renal Stones	Proximal Ureteric Stones	Distal Ureteric Stones
•ESWL	•ESWL	•Conservative management
•PCNL	•Rigid Ureteroscopy	•ESWL
•Flexible Ureteroscopy	•Conservative manegement	•Rigid Ureteroscopy
•Active surveilance		

4. Bladder Pathology

4.1 Bladder Calculi

Bladder stones form due to urinary stasis within the bladder. This stasis can be caused a number of ways including having an obstructing prostate (which can be benign or malignant) or failure of the bladder to empty due to a floppy and weak detrusor muscle. Stones are also common in patients with a long term catheter, the tip of the catheter being a focus of stone formation. In fact patients with a long term catheter in situ have a 25% chance of developing a bladder stone over 5 years.

Bladder stones are more commonly calcium based and can become very large. An ultrasound scan, an X-ray or a flexible cystoscopy can be used to identify bladder stones.

Signs and symptoms of bladder calculi may include	• Pain • Lower urinary tract symptoms (LUTS) • Haematuria • Urinary tract infections • Incidental finding on a scan

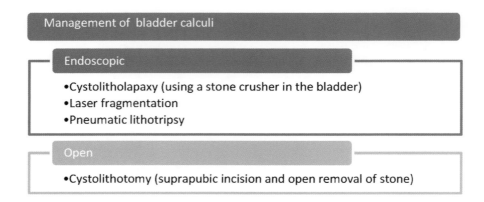

Management of bladder calculi

Endoscopic
- Cystolitholapaxy (using a stone crusher in the bladder)
- Laser fragmentation
- Pneumatic lithotripsy

Open
- Cystolithotomy (suprapubic incision and open removal of stone)

4.2 Bladder Cancer

There are several histological subtypes of bladder cancer. By far the most common is **transitional cell carcinoma (TCC) of the bladder**, however you should also know that squamous cell carcinoma (SCC) and adenocarcinoma of the bladder also exist. Bladder cancer is the 10th most common cancer in the UK. The average age of diagnosis is 73 and it gets more common with age. 10yr survival is approximately 50% for women and 60% for men. However, half of all patients diagnosed with bladder cancer will have non-muscle invasive cancer and the 5 year survival in these patients is 96%.

When taking a history from someone with suspected bladder cancer it is important to think about their risk factors.

4. Bladder Pathology

Risk Factors

Age
- 50-80yrs

Gender
- Male: Female = 2.5 : 1

Ethnicity
- Caucasians at higher risk

Exposure to dyes, rubber, leather, textiles and paint
- **Aromatic amines** which are carcinogenic

SCC risk factors include
- Smoking
- Schistosomiasis
- Chronic cystitis
- Long term catheter
- Intermittent self-catheterisation

Medications
- Including cyclophosphamide and previous pelvic radiotherapy

Smoking

Family history

Genetic conditions such as HNPCC

Signs and symptoms of bladder cancer may include

- Haematuria (often painless and visible, but can also be non-visible)
  - 34% patients >50yrs and 10% of patients <50yrs with macroscopic haematuria have bladder cancer
- Urgency
- Suprapubic/ pelvic mass
- Suprapubic pain
- Recurrent urinary tract infections
- Symptoms of systemic spread

Things to ask in your history:

- Haematuria
  - If so ask your haematuria history as discussed in chapter *2.1*
- Bladder/ abdominal/ Loin pain
  - If so ask your pain history
- LUTS
- Catheter?
- Suffer with UTIs
- Red flag symptoms
- Past medical history
  - Previous urological cancer
  - Radiotherapy
- Family history
- Social history
  - Smoking
  - Occupational exposures
  - Travel

We have already discussed how patients will be investigated for haematuria in chapter *2.1*. All patients with haematuria will need a full set of blood tests, ultrasound or CT and flexible cystoscopy.

A transitional cell carcinoma will look like a papillary lesion within the bladder, often on a stalk which contains its feeding arteries.

Management of Bladder cancer

Psychosocial factors

- Cancer specialist nurse support, lifestyle factors, Macmillan support etc.

Medical

- Radiotherapy
- Chemotherapy (intra-vesical therapy e.g. BCG/Mitomycin C or systemic chemotherapy)
- Palliative (symptomatic relief)

Surgical

- Transurethral resection of bladder tumour (TURBT) is the most common treatment option. A camera endoscope is passed into the bladder via the urethra and diathermy is used to cut the tumour from the inside of the bladder.
- Cystodiathermy or laser (cauterising small lesions within the bladder)
- Cystectomy (removal of the entire bladder for locally advanced bladder cancer)

5. Prostate

5.1 Lower Urinary Tract Symptoms (LUTS)

LUTS are a collection of symptoms which are commonly examined in medical school finals. They are also extremely common and no matter what speciality you work in, you will meet patients suffering with LUTS.

Firstly let's break down a LUTS history. We divide LUTS into **Storage symptoms** and **Voiding symptoms**. Storage symptoms can often be caused by an abnormality of bladder function (its function being to store urine at a low pressure, and to be able to contract when voiding). Whereas voiding symptoms are often caused by an obstruction of bladder outflow (commonly caused by an enlarged prostate or urethral stricture for example). If you take a good LUTS history it can help you to diagnose the cause of the patient's symptoms (and score you high marks in your exams). I have simplified the symptoms in the figure below.

- LUTS (both storage and voiding symptoms are outlined in the green flow-chart below, you will need to ask all of these)
- Haematuria
- Incontinence
- Urinary tract infections
- Haematospermia
- Erectile dysfunction
- Bowel function
- Red Flags
  - Bone/back pain, weight loss, fatigue, night sweats, loss of appetite etc
- Ask about symptoms of cauda equina syndrome to rule this out (as well as with your clinical examination)
- Past medical history
  - Urological malignancy
  - Radiotherapy
  - Previous urological surgery/catheterisation
  - Diabetes or neurological diseases
- Medication history
  - On any treatment for LUTS already?
  - On anti-cholinergics?
  - Diuretics
- Social history
- Family History

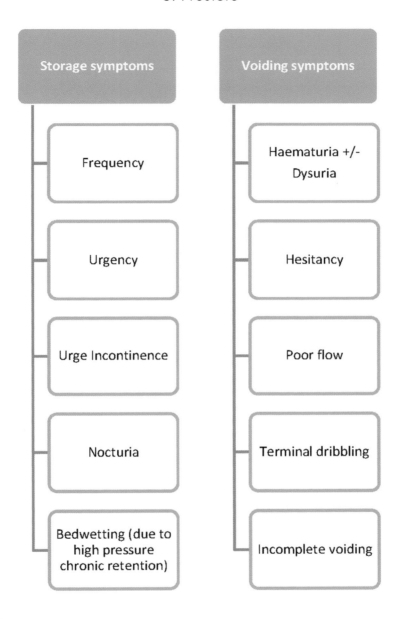

Once you have explored the patients LUTS, you will need to complete a thorough history including red flag symptoms. Examination should include an abdominal examination (making note of any palpable bladder which may be a sign that the patient is not emptying their bladder completely), an examination of the external genitalia (ensure you rule out phimosis or meatal stenosis as a cause) and a digital rectal examination (feeling the size, shape and consistency of the prostate gland).

Other investigations that may be performed to ascertain the cause of these symptoms include:

- Uroflowmetry (the volume of urine passed over time to assess for signs of an over-active bladder, or an obstructive pattern of flow)
- Post-void residual volume of urine within the bladder (using a bladder scanner to see if the patient is in retention)
- PSA and renal function
- Urine dipstick testing and midstream urine sample for culture and sensitivities
- Frequency-volume chart (to monitor fluid input and output for a few consecutive days)
- Consider an ultrasound scan if the residual volume of urine is high or the renal function is impaired to look for signs of hydronephrosis (swollen kidneys)
- Urodynamic testing (to watch how the bladder fills and empties)

Common causes of Voiding LUTS

- Benign prostatic enlargement
- Prostate cancer
- Urethral stricture
- Meatal stenosis
- Phimosis

Common causes of Storage LUTS

- Overactive bladder
- Cystitis or inflammation of the bladder
- Intravesical pathology such as tumour or bladder calculi

Benign Prostatic enlargement

Benign increase in the number of epithelial and stromal cells (hyperplasia) within the prostate gland (also known benign prostatic hyperplasia (BPH)). Often in the transitional zone of the prostate. On digital rectal exam this feels like a **soft enlarged gland**.

Testosterone is converted to its more potent form 'DHT' by 5αReductase. It then binds to receptors inside prostate cells to increase secretions and possibly cell division resulting in gland enlargement.

It is incredibly common and unfortunately most gentlemen will have BPE during the course of their lifetime. However, not everyone will develop LUTS as a result of BPE and the size of the gland doesn't always correlate with the degree of symptoms that a gentleman may experience.

Often LUTS as a result of BPE will progress over time becoming more disruptive until a patient seeks medical attention or develops urinary retention after a trigger event (such as those discussed earlier in chapter *2.2*).

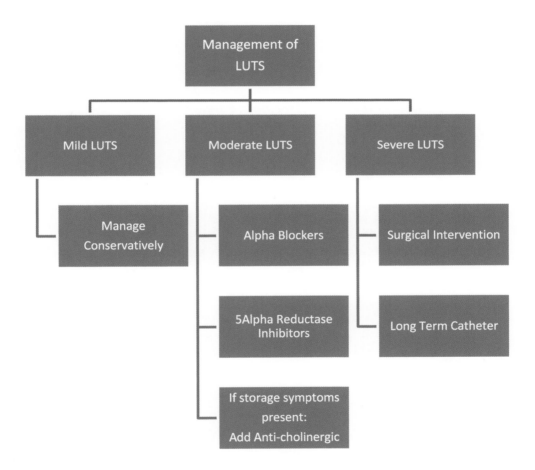

Medical therapy

1) Alpha Blockers (E.g. Tamsulosin)
   - Alpha 1 Adrenoreceptor antagonist that relaxes smooth muscle
   - Side effects include: retrograde ejaculation, dizziness, hypotension

2) 5AlphaReductase Inhibitors (E.g. Finasteride)
   - Inhibits the conversion of testosterone to dihydrotestosterone (DHT) reducing prostatic growth
   - Takes 6 weeks - 6 months to work
   - Side effects include: erectile dysfunction, reduced libido and ejaculation disorders

Surgical options include Transurethral Resection of the Prostate (TURP), Laser prostatectomy, open prostatectomy, prostatic urethral lift, Aquablation etc.

PSA testing

Prostate specific antigen (PSA) is an enzyme produced by prostate to liquefy semen. It can be a very useful indicator of prostate size. However, there are many other factors that can cause a raised PSA (including: urinary tract infections, prostatitis, urinary retention, catheterisation, ejaculation etc.).

PSA levels must therefore be correlated with a digital rectal examination, a good clinical history and examination.

5.2 Prostate Cancer

Adenocarcinoma of the prostate is the most common type of cancer in men in the UK. The management of prostate cancer is an ever-changing field with research making considerable steps forward in recent decades.

Adenocarcinoma of the prostate is multifocal in most instances (80%) and originates in the peripheral zone 75% of the time. This is the reason why prostate cancer can feel like a hard, craggy, irregular gland on digital rectal examination.

Your clinical history should include all of the same questions that are outlined in the orange box in chapter *5.1* LUTS.

Signs and symptoms of Prostate cancer may include	• Lower urinary tract symptoms (LUTS) • Haematospermia (blood in the semen) • Incidentally found with a raised PSA • **Abnormal digital rectal examination (hard, nodular, craggy feeling prostate)** • Bone or back pain (due to metastases) • Signs of metastatic spread

Raised PSA levels will likely prompt a referral for a urology opinion and the patient may be sent for an MRI scan or biopsies of their prostate to rule out a malignant cause of the raised PSA as opposed to BPE. Sometimes we organise a bone scan to check for bony metastases if the PSA is very high.

In order to guide our management options we use the **Gleason grading** system (requires histology from prostate biopsies) to grade the prostate cancer, which allows us to identify low, intermediate and high risk prostate cancers.

The treatment of prostate cancer is very complex and individualised, but to simplify things I have listed some of the possible options below:

Management of Prostate Cancer

Psychosocial factors

- Macmillan support, Cancer Specialist Nurse Support, lifestyle factors, Prostate Cancer UK

Medical

- **Active Surveillance**
  - Suitable for low risk and some intermediate risk cancers if the patient choses to keep a close eye on things and act only if or when the cancer starts to increase in size or become symptomatic.
- **Radiotherapy**
  - Suitable for local and locally advanced cancer as well as for metastatic sites such as in the bones
- **Hormone Therapy**
  - Commonly used for intermediate, high risk and metastatic cancers
- **Chemotherapy**
  - Used in metastatic cancers, especially those which become tolerant to hormone therapy
- **Palliative**
  - Symptomatic relief, which may include a long term catheter, analgesia, radiotherapy to symptomatic sites of metastases and close patient support

Surgical

- Prostatectomy (Open/Laparoscopic/Robotic-assisted)

6. Scrotal Pathology

6.1 Testicular Cancer

Testicular cancer is the most common solid tumour in men 20-45 years of age. There is a lifetime risk of 1 in 210. 99% of men with testicular cancer will survive for 1 year or more and there is a 98% 5-year survival rate.

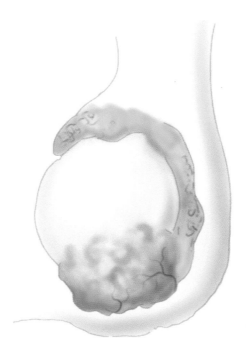

Figure 3: Testicular cancer. Here you can see
a lesion within the body of the testis.

Signs and symptoms of a testicular cancer

- Palpable lump within the testis
- Non-trans illuminable
- May be painful or painless
- Often found on self-examination
- Visualised on Ultrasound scan of the testes

Things to ask in your history:

- Did you notice a lump in the testicle?
- If so when did you first notice this?
- Any change over time?
- Is it painful/tender?
- Dysuria
- LUTS
- Penile discharge
- Recent unprotected sexual contact
- Trauma
- History of subfertility
- Red Flag symptoms
  - Haemoptysis, Bone/back pain, weight loss, fatigue, night sweats, loss of appetite etc
- Past medical history
  - Previous testicular cancer
  - Cryptorchidism (see chapter *6.2*)
  - HIV
- Family history

6. Scrotal Pathology

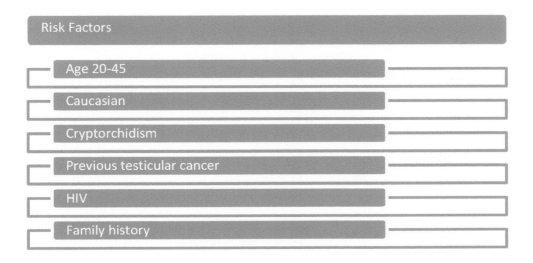

Risk Factors

- Age 20-45
- Caucasian
- Cryptorchidism
- Previous testicular cancer
- HIV
- Family history

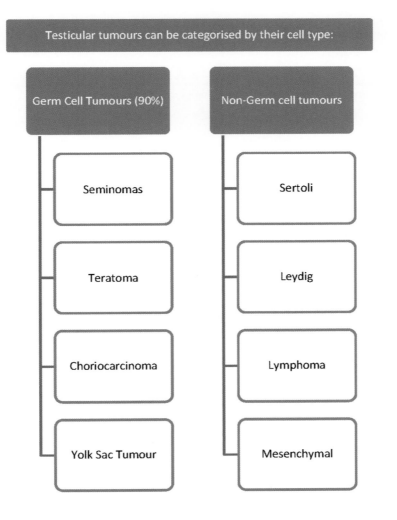

Testicular tumours can be categorised by their cell type:

Germ Cell Tumours (90%)
- Seminomas
- Teratoma
- Choriocarcinoma
- Yolk Sac Tumour

Non-Germ cell tumours
- Sertoli
- Leydig
- Lymphoma
- Mesenchymal

How do we investigate a possible testicular tumour?

1) Urgent ultrasound scan of the testes
2) Chest X-ray (if symptomatic for pulmonary metastases)
3) Tumour Markers (not always raised and not diagnostic but can be useful to check response before vs. after-surgery)
   - α Fetoprotein (AFP)
   - Human chorionic gonadotropin (hCG)
   - Lactate dehydrogenase (LDH)

Management of Testicular Cancer

Semen cryopreservation

- To be considered for patients whom have not yet completed their family

Urgent radical **inguinal** orchidectomy

- Performed via an inguinal incision avoiding the risk of seeding tumour on the way out of the scrotum

Testicular prosthesis

- Depending on the wishes of the patient

Treatment for Metastatic disease

- Retroperitoneal lymph node dissection if the tumour has metastasised to the lymph nodes (testicles drain to their embryological origin i.e. the para-aortic lymph nodes)
- Chemotherapy
- Radiotherapy

6.2 Undescended Testes (Cryptorchidism)

Boys born at term should have both testes within the scrotum (which is examined during a newborn baby check). Pre-term boys have a higher chance of having undescended testes, though most of these will descend within the first 3 months.

> **Untreated undescended testes increase a patient's risk of:**
>
> • Infertility
> • Testicular torsion
> • Testicular cancer (cryptorchidism does not technically increase one's risk of cancer, but as the testicles are not examinable patients that go on to develop cancer present later)

Undescended testes can be described clinically as:

• **Palpable**
• **Impalpable**

We can also describe them anatomically as:

• **Maldescended** (testes that lie somewhere along the normal path of descent, this is the most common presentation)
• **Ectopic** (often lying in the thigh, perineum or in the opposite side of the scrotum)

If the testicle can be easily brought down into the scrotum on examination, this is deemed a '**Retractile**' testis. This is a variant of normal and often does not require surgical intervention. However, both patients and healthcare workers must remain vigilant with these as there is a risk of progression to an **Ascending** testicle which would require treatment.

Ascending testes are seen later in childhood, in boys who have had testes within the scrotum previously. Orchidopexy is recommended to reduce the risk of infertility, testicular cancer and allow for easy self examination.

Impalpable testes can be found at the following locations:

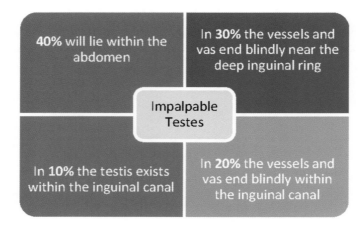

Where the vessels and vas end blindly the testis no longer exists. The most likely cause of this is intrauterine testicular torsion.

Note: If there are bilateral impalpable testes, Karyotype testing is recommended.

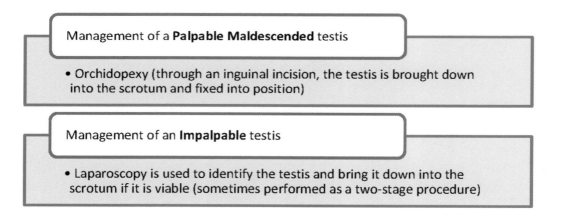

6.3 Lumps and Bumps

In most cases if you are presented with a testicular or scrotal lump in your finals it will be focussing on the clinical examination of the lump. Plastic models exist which simulate the presence of different testicular and scrotal pathology, but you could also be expected to take a clinical history from a patient or an actor before proceeding to examine the model. In clinical practise it is essential that you take a thorough clinical history as this may drastically change your differential diagnosis (for example changing your suspicion as to whether a lump may be malignant or not).

Things to ask in your history:

- When did you first notice this?
- Any change over time?
- Is it painful/tender? (if so full pain history)
- Fever
- Dysuria
- LUTS
- Penile discharge
- Recent unprotected sexual contact
- Trauma
- History of subfertility
- Red Flag symptoms
- Past medical history
  - Previous testicular cancer
  - Cryptorchidism (see chapter **6.2**)
  - HIV
- Family history

How to describe a lump on examination?

It's easy in the heat of the moment in exams to forget what to mention when you find a lump on examination of the external genitalia, here's a helpful way of remembering things:

It takes **6 S**tudents, **5 C**linicians and **4 t**eachers to describe a lump.

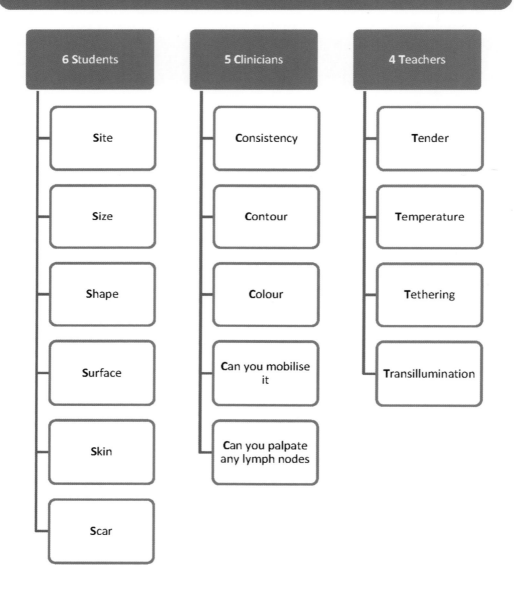

6 Students	5 Clinicians	4 Teachers
Site	**C**onsistency	**T**ender
Size	**C**ontour	**T**emperature
Shape	**C**olour	**T**ethering
Surface	**C**an you mobilise it	**T**ransillumination
Skin	**C**an you palpate any lymph nodes	
Scar		

Hydrocele

Is an accumulation of fluid within the tunica vaginalis. These can be primary or secondary (a sign of malignancy, trauma, infection or torsion for example). They can be non-communicating (typical in adults) or communicating with the peritoneum (due to a patent processus vaginalis, these can change in size when standing vs lying down due to increased intra-abdominal pressure).

Signs and symptoms of a hydrocele	•Fluctuant scrotal swelling •Transilluminable swelling •Unable to palpate the testis separate from the swelling •Can get above the swelling (to rule out a hernia)

A non-communicating hydrocele is often caused by either increased production of fluid by the tunica vaginalis, reduced resorption of fluid or impairment in lymphatic drainage.

Treatment options include: conservative management, surgical repair, or aspiration if a patient is not suitable for an anaesthetic.

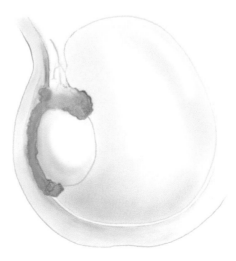

Figure 4: Hydrocele. Here you can see an accumulation of fluid within the tunica vaginalis.

Varicocele

Dilatation of the testicular veins which can be unilateral or bilateral.

Signs and symptoms of varicocele

- Feels like a 'bag of worms'
- Patient may feel a dragging sensation in the area
- Can cause aching
- Identified on Ultrasound scan of the testes

Be aware of new left sided varicoceles in adults. As mentioned previously in chapter *3.2* renal cancers that involve the left renal vein can cause obstruction of the left spermatic vein causing a left sided varicocele. Whereas the right testicular vein drains directly into IVC.

Treatment options include: conservative management, surgical ligation or embolisation.

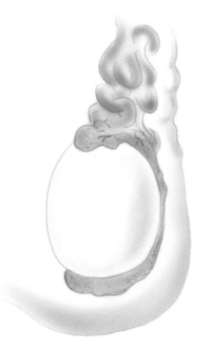

Figure 5: Varicocele. Here you can see dilatation of the testicular veins.

Epididymal Cyst

As the name suggests it is a cyst of the epididymis. These can be either symptomatic or asymptomatic and can vary greatly in size. They are fluctuant swellings that are separate from the body of the testis. They are sometimes transilluminable on examination and can be easily confirmed on ultrasound scan.

Signs and symptoms of epididymal cysts	• Palpable lump(s) within the epididymis • Difficult to trans illuminate • May be painful or painless • Visualised on Ultrasound scan of the testes

Treatment options include: conservative management or surgical excision if large or symptomatic.

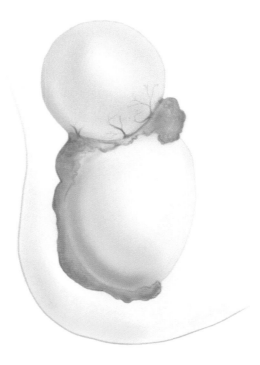

Figure 6: Epididymal cyst. Here you can see an accumulation of fluid within the epididymis.

63

Sebaceous cyst of the scrotum

These cysts are hard, often containing a whitish-yellow coloured substance.

Signs and symptoms of scrotal sebaceous cysts	• Palpable lump(s) within the scrotal skin • Lumps are tethered to the skin and are separate to the underlying testis and epididymis • Lumps feel rubbery • Non-trans illuminable • Often multiple cysts • Usualy painless unless infected

Treatment options include: conservative management or surgical excision.

6.4 Epididymo-orchitis

A common acute urological presentation but one that is often difficult to differentiate from a torted testicle. Epididymo-orchitis is infection of the epididymis and/or testicle. Causative organisms are often those causing urinary tract infections such as *E.Coli* that have tracked along the vas deferens, but you must also rule out a sexually transmitted infection such as *Chlamydia* or *Gonorrhoea* as a cause. Mumps used to be a common cause of orchitis in boys but this is now thankfully rare due to the MMR vaccine. Nonetheless you should examine the parotid glands for signs of parotitis in all patients presenting with epididymo-orchitis.

If left untreated the patient can become septic and develop an abscess. On-going infection can cause chronic testicular pain and can result in necrosis of the testicle.

6. Scrotal Pathology

Symptoms

- May have preceding symptoms of a urinary tract infection
- LUTS
- Penile discharge
- Painful hemiscrotum
- Feverish

Signs

- A hot, swollen and erythematous hemiscrotum
- Testicle and epididymis very tender to touch
- Epididymis and cord may feel thickened

Things to ask in your history:

- Time of onset of pain?
- Has it changed over time?
- Any radiation of pain?
- Full pain history (see pain history box below)
- Trauma?
- History of similar episodes?
- Recent unprotected sexual intercourse?
- Sexual health history
- Penile discharge?
- Dysuria?
- Fever?
- LUTS discussed in chapter *5.1*
- Urinary tract infections
- Recent instrumentation/catheterisation of the urinary tract?
- Urological history or previous scrotal surgery?

Management of Epididymo-orchitis

- First you must rule out torsion of the testicle and escalate the case to the urologist on call immediately.

- The management of epididymo-orchitis will largely depend on the history you have taken from the patient.

- If a sexually-transmitted infection is likely and the patient is younger (less than 40 years of age) then the patient will require a full STI screen prior to starting them on antibiotics (such as Ceftriaxone and Doxycycline for example) to cover *Chlamydia* or *Gonorrhoea*).

- If a urinary tract infection is the likely cause then antibiotics are used that will cover organisms such as *E.Coli* and have good penetration in the testis and epididymis e.g. Ciprofloxacin.

- Courses of antibiotics for epididymo-orchitis are usually given for 10-14 days followed by either a review of the patient by either their General practitioner or the Urology team.

7. Penile Pathology

7.1 Erectile Dysfunction

> "The recurrent inability to achieve or maintain an erection inhibiting sexual intercourse."

This is often a multifactorial condition that can be largely attributed to both psychogenic and organic causes. Organic causes are more likely to present in patients with other health problems and often have a gradual onset with no significant loss of libido.

Things to ask in your history:

- When did it first start?
- Is it getting progressively worse?
- Able to achieve an erection? If so, how long for
- Able to achieve penetrative sexual intercourse?
- Presence of morning tumescence
- Loss of libido
- PMH: Diabetes, hypertension, vascular disease, neurological conditions, pelvic surgery or radiotherapy
- Rx: What treatments have they tried already?
- Social: Drugs, alcohol and smoking
- Psychosocial: relationship status and difficulties, anxieties, depression

Things to examine:

- Cardiovascular examination
- Neurological examination
- Examination of the abdomen
- Examine external genitalia (Look for deformity, shortening, secondary sexual characteristics, testicular atrophy)
- Digital rectal examination

Investigations

Blood tests

- Testosterone, Luteinising hormone (LH) and Follicle-stimulating hormone (FSH), Prolactin, Sex hormone-binding globulin, Thyroid function tests (TFTs) and glucose levels.

Nocturnal penile tumescence testing

- Rings are placed over the penis to measure frequency and duration of spontaneous erections overnight. If erections are proven, this can lead to the diagnosis of psychogenic erectile dysfunction

Imaging

- MRI scans can assess for Peyronie's plaques. Doppler Ultrasound scans can be used to assess vasculature. Neither of which are routinely performed but can be used in specific cases.

7. Penile Pathology

Organic Causes of ED

Endocrine

- Diabetes Mellitus/Metabolic syndrome
- Hyper/hypothyroidism
- Hyperprolactinaemia
- Hypogonadism

Neurogenic

- Spinal cord pathology (e.g. Spina bifida, cord compression)
- Multiple sclerosis
- Parkinson's disease

Vascular

- Hyperlipidaemia
- Peripheral vascular disease
- Hypertension

Medication

- Anti-depressants
- Parkinsons Medications
- Anti Androgens
- Anti hypertensives

Miscellaneous

- Alcohol
- Smoking
- Pelvic surgery
- Pelvic radiotherapy
- Peyronie's disease
- Substance abuse

Management of Erectile Dysfunction

Psychogenic ED

- Psychosexual therapy

Organic ED

- Phosphodiesterase type-5 (PDE5) inhibitors
  - Block the breakdown of cGMP by phosphodiesterase to cause vasodilation in cavernosal smooth muscle. Still requires sexual stimulation.
- Intraurethral Prostaglandins
  - Increases cAMP intracavernosally resulting in vasodilation.
- Intracavernosal injection therapy
  - Injected by the patient intracavernosally.
- Vacuum erection device
  - Patients are trained to use a vacuum pump device.
- Testosterone replacement therapy
  - Used to treat hypogonadism.
- Penile Prosthesis
  - A range of prostheses are now available and are inserted at specialist hospitals.

7.2 Peyronie's disease

> "Curvature of the penis caused by the development of fibrotic tissue on the tunica albuginea."

A benign condition that becomes more common with age. There is an initial inflammatory phase characterised by increasing deformity of the penis and painful erections followed by the quiescent phase during which the deformity stabilises.

The exact cause is unknown but it is thought that repeated minor trauma causes microvascular damage during intercourse, resulting in inflammation and fibrosis in genetically predisposed men.

It is associated with diabetes, hypertension, high cholesterol, Dupuytren's contracture and plantar fasciitis.

Things to ask in your history:

- When did it first start?
- Is it getting progressively worse? Or has it plateaued in severity?
- Able to achieve an erection?
- Is it painful?
- What is the angle of the penis when erect?
- Have you experienced penile shortening?
- Able to achieve penetrative sexual intercourse?
- Subfertility?
- Trauma?
- PMH: Liver disease, Dupuytren's contracture, plantar fasciitis, hypertension, vascular disease, urological surgery, connective tissue disorders
- Social history
- Psychosocial: relationship status and difficulties, anxieties, depression
- Family history

Signs and symptoms of
Peyronie's diesease

- A significant curvature to the penis, usually only notable when erect
- Penile shortening
- Penile pain
- Erectile dysfunction
- Difficulty having penetrative intercourse
- A palpable fibrous plaque (or several) along the shaft of the penis at the site of angular deviation
- Altered shape of the penis due to fibrous plaque formation (can have an hour-glass appearance with a tight fibrous band at the shaft)

Management of Peyronie's disease

Medical

- Oral pentoxifyline, verapamil injections, extra-corporeal shockwave therapy or vacuum tumescence and penile traction devices all have limited evidence.

Surgical

- Surgical correction will only be performed on stable plaques and may include Nesbit's procedure, Lue procedure, plication procedures or the insertion of a penile prosthesis.

7.3 Phimosis

"A tight foreskin (prepuce) which is unable to retract over the glans."

This is usually asymptomatic but patients may notice ballooning of the foreskin on micturition. This can also cause pain and irritation during sexual intercourse and men may develop infections of the foreskin and glans (balanoposthitis).

Things to ask in your history:

- When did you first notice that the foreskin was tight?
- Able to retract it?
- Difficulty passing urine?
- Ballooning of the foreskin on micturition?
- Balanoposthitis? (infection)
- Pain on erections?
- Difficulty having penetrative intercourse?
- Past medical history
  - Previous urological surgery
  - Diabetes
- Medication
  - Tried steroid creams?
- Social history

Balanitis Xerotica Obliterans (BXO) is a chronic inflammatory condition (seen as the male equivalent of lichen sclerosus) that can cause phimosis. Chronic inflammation results in the development of a fibrous, tight foreskin often with grey/white discoloration, it can cause urethral stenosis and can be associated with penile cancer. Steroids can be applied topically in the first instance but often a circumcision is required.

Phimosis is normal (otherwise called physiological phimosis) in childhood and almost all (99%) foreskins are retractile by the age of 16.

The gold standard of treatment for phimosis is a **circumcision** (excision of the foreskin). As well as removing the phimotic foreskin, there is evidence to suggest that circumcision may also reduce one's risk of sexually transmitted infections and penile cancer.

7.4 Urethral stricture disease

> "Subepithelial fibrosis within the corpus spongiosum causing a narrowing of the urethra."

These can be caused by trauma e.g. straddle injuries, iatrogenic (including catheterisation and instrumentation) and can also likely be caused by inflammation e.g. urethritis.

Signs and symptoms of Urethral stricture diesease

- Voiding LUTS (may be complicated by storage LUTS as well)
- Urinary retention
- May experience urinary tract infections
- Risk factors may aid clinical suspicion
- Difficult to pass a catheter, may hit resistance or obstruction distal to the prostate

Things to ask in your history:

- LUTS (storage and voiding symptoms as outlined in the green flow-chart in chapter **5.1**)
- Urinary tract infections
- Sexually transmitted infections
- Incontinence
- Red flag symptoms
- Past medical history
  - Urological surgery
  - Previous catheterisation
  - Radiotherapy
- Medication history
- Social history
- Family History

Treatment of these is to perform sequential *urethral dilatation* in theatre, or to incise the stricture with an endoscopic knife (*optical urethrotomy*). Following these operations patients are often taught how to perform *Intermittent self-dilatation* (ISD) of the urethra to try and prevent the stricture from progressing again. If the stricture continues to return, patients may require incision of the stricture and Urethroplasty (urethral reconstruction).

8. Incontinence

Incontinence is a common presentation in urology. The prevalence of incontinence in the population is 30% with females being twice as likely to develop incontinence as men.

Risk Factors

- Age
- Gender
- Oestrogen deficiency
- Anatomical disorders (e.g. Fistulae)
- Childbirth and pregnancy
- Abdominal, pelvic, perineal and prostate surgery
- Diabetes
- Smoking
- Obesity
- Urinary tract infections
- Poor mobility
- Neurological disorders
  - E.g. Multiple sclerosis, Parkinson's disease, spinal cord Injury etc.

- Duration of symptoms
- Change over time
- Timing of incontinence
  - Continuous
  - At specific times e.g. with an increase in intra-abdominal pressure (coughing, sneezing, laughing etc)
- Associated symptoms
  - Urgency
  - Frequency
  - Dysuria
  - Bladder pain
- Use of incontinence pads? If so how many per day/night
- Use of containment devices e.g. convene or catheter
- Bladder diary (discuss fluid intake habits including timing of drinking, alcohol and caffeine)
- Obstetric history for female patients
- Post-menopausal?
- Rule out cauda-equina (in combination with examination findings)
- Bowel function
- Sexual dysfunction
- Psychosocial impact of symptoms
- Past medical history
  - Previous urological or gynaecological surgery
  - Pelvic radiotherapy
  - COPD
  - Neurological disorders
- Medication history
- Social history
  - Smoking
  - Alcohol
- Family History

Always assess the impact that these symptoms have on the patient's life. It is very important that we discover the cause of a patient's incontinence in order to address it. It is not uncommon to hear that a patient with incontinence is too scared to leave the home as they worry about having an accident in public. Incontinence can have a devastating impact on an individual's quality of life.

A full systematic examination is required including an abdominal examination, examination of the external genitalia, digital rectal examination (remember to check sphincter power), lower limb neurological examination and a pelvic examination in females.

8.1 Stress Urinary Incontinence (SUI)

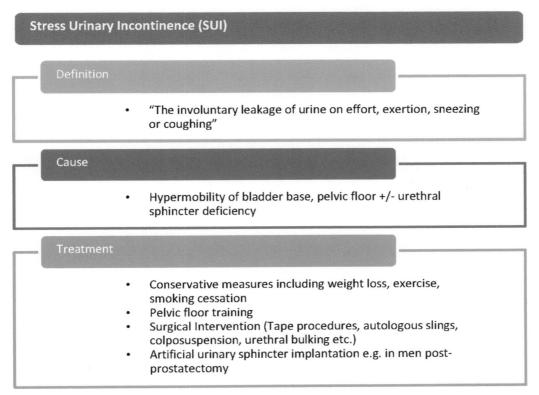

Stress Urinary Incontinence (SUI)

Definition
- "The involuntary leakage of urine on effort, exertion, sneezing or coughing"

Cause
- Hypermobility of bladder base, pelvic floor +/- urethral sphincter deficiency

Treatment
- Conservative measures including weight loss, exercise, smoking cessation
- Pelvic floor training
- Surgical Intervention (Tape procedures, autologous slings, colposuspension, urethral bulking etc.)
- Artificial urinary sphincter implantation e.g. in men post-prostatectomy

8.2 Urge Urinary Incontinence (UUI)

Urge Urinary Incontinence (UUI)

Definition

- "The involuntary leakage of urine accompanied by or immediately proceeded by urgency (a sudden strong desire to void)"

Cause

- Over active detrusor muscle

Over Active Bladder Syndrome

- "Urgency with or without urge incontinence, often with frequency and nocturia"

Treatment

- Conservative measures (reduce caffeine, alcohol, biofeedback, electrical stimulation)
- Anti-muscarinic medication e.g. Oxybutynin = detrusor relaxation
- B-3 adrenoreceptor agonist - Mirabegron
- Neuromodulation (sacral nerve stimulator or percutaneous tibial nerve stimulation)
- Botox (injected into the bladder wall using a cystoscope)
- Clam cystoplasty or Urinary diversion

8.3 Mixed Urinary Incontinence (MUI)

Mixed Urinary Incontinence (MUI)

Definition

- "The involuntary leakage of urine associated with effort, exertion, coughing or sneezing accompanied by or immediately proceeded by urgency (a sudden strong desire to void)"

Cause

- Hypermobility of bladder base, pelvic floor +/- urethral sphincter deficiency AND Over active detrusor muscle

8.4 Overflow Incontinence

Overflow Incontinence

Definition

- "The involuntary leakage of urine when the bladder is abnormally distended with large volumes of urine"

Cause

- Often due to bladder outflow obstruction (men with chronic retention) and a degree of detrusor failure

Management

- Treat bladder outflow obstruction
- Long term catheter
- Intermittent self-catheterisation

9. Urinary Tract Infections

9.1 Urinary Tract Infections

Inflammation of the urinary tract following bacterial invasion. Infection of the bladder is otherwise known as *Cystitis* and infection of the Kidney and upper tracts (associated with fever, loin pain, nausea and vomiting) is also called *Pyelonephritis*.

The best way to break these down is to separate infections into 2 categories:

Uncomplicated UTI

- In an otherwise normal urinary tract.

Complicated UTI

- One occurring in an abnormal or male urinary tract. This may be either a structurally abnormal tract e.g. bladder outflow obstruction or a fistula, or this may be a urinary tract that contains an abnormality e.g. cancer or stones.

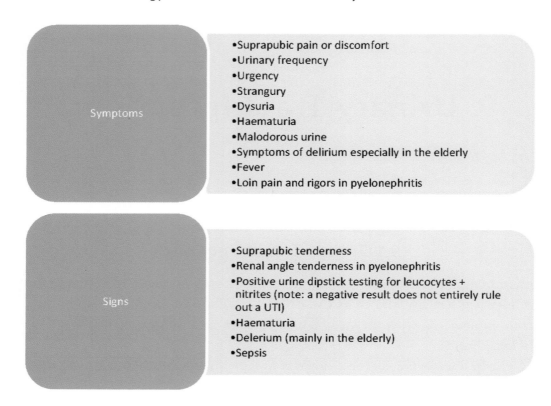

Symptoms
- Suprapubic pain or discomfort
- Urinary frequency
- Urgency
- Strangury
- Dysuria
- Haematuria
- Malodorous urine
- Symptoms of delirium especially in the elderly
- Fever
- Loin pain and rigors in pyelonephritis

Signs
- Suprapubic tenderness
- Renal angle tenderness in pyelonephritis
- Positive urine dipstick testing for leucocytes + nitrites (note: a negative result does not entirely rule out a UTI)
- Haematuria
- Delerium (mainly in the elderly)
- Sepsis

- When did the symptoms start?
- Any change over time?
- Taken any courses of antibiotics already?
- LUTS
- Dysuria
- Haematuria
- Previous UTIs, if so how many and how often
- Precipitating factors? E.g. sexual intercourse
- Catheter in situ?
- Post-menopause?
- Bowel function
- Fluid Intake
- Red flag symptoms
- Past medical history
  - Stones, cancer, diabetes, neurological disorders, HIV
- Medication history
  - Details on courses of antibiotics including how many courses, which antibiotics and what duration
  - Immunosuppressants
- Social history
  - Smoking
  - Occupation

Mid-stream urine (MSU) sampling

Always send an MSU sample in cases of a suspected UTI. Bacteria in the urine (*Bacteriuria*) may be either symptomatic or asymptomatic. Asymptomatic bacteriuria is very common especially in the elderly and does not necessarily require treatment. If there are white blood cells in the urine (*Pyuria*) as well as bacteria, this is often a sign of an inflammatory response in the urinary tract and is likely to require antibiotic therapy. Note that whilst urine dipstick testing can be useful in adding diagnostic value when seeing patients with symptomatic UTI's, a negative urine dipstick does not rule out a urinary tract infection.

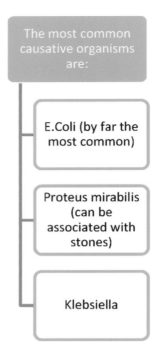

For uncomplicated UTI's in women a 3 day course of oral antibiotics or a single dose of fosfomycin will normally clear the infection. A complicated infection will often require a 7 day course of antibiotics, and may require intravenous (IV) antibiotics if the patient is systemically unwell.

Risk Factors for UTI's
Female
Previous UTI's
Post-menopausal
Age
Diabetes
Pregancy
Anatomical abnormalities of the urinary tract
Catheters

9.2 Recurrent UTI's

Defined as more than 2 infections in 6 months, or 3 within a year. This can be caused by *bacterial re-infection* (UTI's caused by different bacteria) or by *bacterial persistence* (repeat infections by the same organism). This can also occur if a UTI has been inadequately treated (*unresolved infection*).

Recurrent UTI's should always be thoroughly investigated for an alternative cause such as urinary tract stones or malignancy (by upper tract imaging with either a CT or Ultrasound scan and by cystoscopy). Once a sinister cause has been excluded the infections can be treated in a step-wise manner:

Management of Recurrent UTI's

Conservative measures

- Increase fluid intake
- Optimise blood sugars if diabetic
- Vaginal Oestrogens in post-menopausal women
- Avoid constipation
- Good hygiene
- Voiding before and after sexual intercourse
- Avoid bubble bath and bath salts
- Avoid spermicides
- D-mannose (available from health food shops)
- Cranberry juice/tablets (limited evidence for its use)

Self-start Antibiotics

- When a patient feels that they have developed a new UTI, they will have a short course of antibiotics stored at home to start immediately.

Post-coital prophylactic antibiotics

- Patients can take one dose of prophylactic antibiotics following sexual intercourse if this is a consistent trigger for UTI's.

Long-term low dose prophylactic antibiotics

- Often started according to previous MSU culture and sensitivities. Antibiotics can be stopped after 3-6 months to see whether the bacteria have been fully eradicated.

10. Practical tips for Junior doctors

Male catheterisation:

Understanding the anatomy or the urethra will help when struggling with a catheter. When first inserting a catheter in a male make sure you have a good grasp of the penis and lift the penis up at a 45-degree angle to the supine body. This will straighten the urethra. Insert the catheter until you feel it bounce off the prostate, then lower the penis until it is almost at the same level of the body, this will help the catheter slip through the prostate and into the bladder. Twisting the catheter gently between your fingertips on insertion can also help it to pass through the prostate.

The 2 most common reasons for failing to catheterise a man are:

1. **An enlarged prostate**
2. **A urethral stricture.**

> 1. **An enlarged prostate**: Here you are able to advance approximately half of the catheter into the urethra before it bounces off the prostate and will go no further. In these circumstances, try a catheter with a **larger** diameter, as these are less likely to cause a false passage and are a little sturdier for you to push in.
>
> If you are still unable to pass a catheter it is time to call a senior for help, who may elect to try a Tiemann-tip or Coudé-tip catheter

(catheters with a little bend at the tip) which may help in getting around the prostate.

If your senior is unable to insert a catheter, call the Urologist on call. They may need to insert a catheter using a flexible cystoscope for guidance or a supra-pubic catheter may need to be inserted.

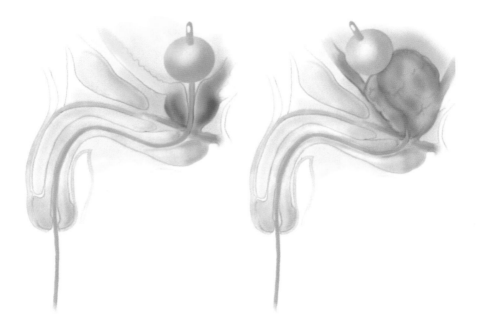

Figure 7: An enlarged prostate. Here you can see how prostatic enlargement can significantly alter the path of the urethra making catheterisation more challenging.

2. **A urethral stricture** may become evident when you are only able to advance the catheter a little way into the urethra. In these cases, try a silicone catheter with a **smaller** diameter enabling you to pass the tube through the narrowing in the urethra.

If you and your senior have been unable to insert a catheter, call the Urologist on call. They may need to insert a catheter using a flexible cystoscope for guidance, urethral dilatation may be required, or a supra-pubic catheter may need to be inserted.

Consider providing prophylactic antibiotic cover for catheterisation (E.g. Gentamicin or Ciprofloxacin) if:

- Previous infections from catheterisation

- High risk of infection

- Difficult insertion

- Those at risk of endocarditis

Lubricating gel

When putting lubricating gel such as Instillagel or Hydrocaine in, hold the penis up and push the gel in very slowly. Use more than one gel if it is a difficult catheterisation. Don't rush, clamp urethra gently between finger and thumb to give it time to work. Taking time for the installagel to work will allow the lidocaine to take effect and will also relax the patient a little, causing them less distress, making it easier for you.

Female catheterisation

Female catheterisation is far easier, however many nurses are trained to do this, so often the first one you will be asked to insert is for a patient whom several nurses have already attempted unsuccessfully to catheterise (which is a little daunting). So ask for some help from the nurse looking after the patient and maybe another pair of hands to assist in passing you equipment. Good positioning is key, the woman needs to be in the smear position, but if you are struggling to locate the urethra you can try with the patient in the left lateral position.

The three most common reasons for failing to catheterise a female are:

1. **Meatal Stenosis**
2. **Cystocele**
3. **Position of the urethral meatus (may lie in the anterior wall of the vagina)**

1. **Meatal stenosis** will present as a very tight urethra. Most of the time you are still able to pass a catheter so don't panic. Find a small diameter, long term catheter, as these are more likely to pass the stenosis and are a little more rigid. If you still struggle, call your senior.

2. **Cystocele:** You may struggle to see the urethra if there is an anterior wall prolapse, or you may be able to insert the catheter only a little way into the urethra. If this is the case, try reducing the prolapse by pushing the anterior wall of the vagina anteriorly to return the urethra to its normal position.

When consenting a patient for catheterisation you must ensure the patient understands the possible risks, complications, benefits and alternatives. Risks of catheterisation include:

Acute risks of catheterisation

- Pain
- Bleeding
- False passage
- Failure
- Urethral damage
- Paraphimosis
- Infection
  - 100% of catheters are colonised by bacteria at one week
  - 5% risk of catheter related sepsis per day
  - 8% bacteraemia

Chronic risks of catheterisation

- Stricture formation
- Failed TWOC
- Stones
- Cancer

Short Term catheters are PTFE Coated Latex and can remain in situ for a maximum of 4 weeks. Long Term catheters are Silicone and should be changed at least every 12 weeks.

The commonly used sizes of adult catheters range from 12-24Fr. The sizes you are most likely to encounter on a general ward range from 12-16Fr.

3-way Catheters

These are generally a little wider bore than 2-way catheters. They have 3 distal ends to the catheter: one for inflating the balloon, one to insert irrigating fluids into the bladder and the last is the outflow. Consider inserting a 3-way catheter in patients with haematuria to allow for continuous irrigation and bladder washouts. Balloons of 3-way catheters can be filled with up to 20mL water although 10ml are usually enough to hold any catheter in place.

Finally, a few key things to remember when catheterising a patient:

ALWAYS:

- Measure the residual volume of urine that drains after insertion
- Document the volume of sterile water in the balloon
- Document the consent, procedure details and findings in the notes
- Replace the foreskin to original position in gentlemen

NEVER:

- Use a female catheter in a male
- Force the catheter – you may create a false passage
- Inflate the balloon before urine is draining

Suprapubic Catheters

You will at some stage in your career be asked to change a suprapubic catheter...don't panic, they are even easier to change than a urethral catheter. The tract is very short and a lot easier to negotiate than a male urethra.

Unless they have been inserted for the first time within the last 3 months (in which case it will need to be changed by the urology team) you will be able to change it using normal catheterisation equipment.

Get everything ready and have an assistant with you for the first few times you change a suprapubic catheter. Replace it with the same type and size of catheter but have a smaller catheter handy just in case you struggle. Take note of how much of the original catheter was inside the bladder to avoid inserting the new catheter too far (if you insert too much it may enter the urethra). When inserting the replacement catheter, use the same trajectory that the old catheter had to avoid missing the tract. NEVER attempt to insert a NEW suprapubic catheter yourself, this is a job for the Urology doctor on-call. Remember, if this is the first time it is being changed since insertion – call the Urologist on call.

Removing catheters

Most of the time this is simple, you deflate the balloon and gently pull the catheter out. However, on occasion you may struggle to deflate the balloon. On these occasions you can try pushing a further 10mls of sterile water into the balloon (stopping immediately if this causes the patient discomfort). Often this will help unblock the balloon; you can then deflate it by removing the total volume of water in the balloon.

Bladder washouts

These are commonly performed to remove clots from a bladder, and you may be asked to perform this. Flushing a catheter can also unblock a catheter that has stopped draining.

Equipment required:

- 50ml bladder syringe
- Bladder irrigation fluid
- Large bowl
- Personal protective equipment

How to perform Bladder washout on the ward:

1. Ensure that a 3-way catheter has been inserted
2. Stop and disconnect the irrigation fluid
3. Measure bladder volume with bladder scanner
4. Place the end of the catheter in a bowl
5. Wipe ports down with alcohol wipe
6. Squeeze irrigation fluid into irrigation port of catheter using a 50ml bladder syringe
7. Take note of how much you put in
8. Take note of how much comes out, what colour, are there clots?
9. If it is not freely draining you can try gently pulling back on syringe
10. Do not keep putting more in if none comes out – as this will become painful
11. In this case the patient may need a change of catheter or to go to theatre for cystoscopy and bladder washout, discuss this with the Urology team
12. Ask Surgical/Urology nurses for help – they are very experienced.

Flushing a Nephrostomy

A blocked nephrostomy is a common reason for acute admission to hospital. Patients often present with flank/ back pain and reduced nephrostomy output.

Take a full history and examine the patient to rule out other problems. Take bloods to check for infection and discuss with your senior or the Urology team.

How to flush a blocked nephrostomy:

1. Do it under supervision of senior
2. Similar to bladder washout
3. Aseptic technique
4. Slowly instil 2-5ml Normal Saline and do not aspirate
5. If it remains blocked – discuss with your senior immediately

11. References and further reading

Reynard, J., Brewster, S., & Biers, S. (2013-02). Oxford Handbook of Urology 3rd Edition. Oxford, UK: Oxford University Press. ISBN 9780199696130.

Alan J. Wein & Louis R. Kavoussi & Alan W. Partin & Craig A. Peters. Campbell-Walsh Urology, 11th Edition. Elsevier 2016. ISBN 9781455775675.

David FM. Thomas, Patrick G. Duffy and Anthony MK. Rickwood. Essentials of Paediatric Urology, 2nd Edition. Informa Healthcare 2008. ISBN 9781841846330.

Smith and Tanagho's General Urology 18th Edition.Lange, McGraw-Hill 2013. ISBN 9780071632607.

Resuscitation council UK. Advanced Life Support 7th Edition. Feb 2016. ISBN 9781903812303

https://www.cancerresearchuk.org/

https://www.baus.org.uk/

https://uroweb.org/

###

Congratulations, you made it to the end of the book!

Thank you for reading.

I am extremely proud of this textbook; it took over 3 years to write with the help of the extremely dedicated editing team. I sincerely hope that you have found it useful. It would be very helpful if you could leave a review and please do tell your colleagues about it, afterall the only way to improve healthcare is to work as a team.

I look forward to working with you all.

Ricky Ellis

Index

Author Biography

Ricky Ellis is a Urology Specialist Registrar working in the East Midlands, United Kingdom. He is also a Research Fellow for the Intercollegiate Committee for Basic Surgical Examinations (ICBSE), undertaking research with the aim of improving medical education, examinations and selection methods.

Ricky organises Urology teaching courses including the 'Urology Boot Camp for Medical Students', which was recently nominated for several excellence awards. He is passionate about improving training for medical students and junior doctors.

What little spare time he has he mostly spends with his family, his dog and playing sport.

Printed in Great Britain
by Amazon